Balance Exercise for Seniors Over 60

10-Minute Illustrated, Easy-to-Follow Exercise to Empower Your Golden Years, to Prevent Fall and Improve Stability. With a 21-day Workout plan.

Vitali Aging

**BELOW IS YOUR BONUS EBOOK
TITLED: ANTI-INFLAMMATORY DIET
FOR SENIORS**

**SCAN THE QR CODE TO
DOWNLOAD**

Table of Content

Introduction

Introduction

Maintaining balance is a fundamental aspect of overall well-being, particularly as we age. As the years advance, the body undergoes natural changes, impacting coordination and stability. The question then arises: how can individuals in their 60s and beyond cultivate and enhance their balance? Exercise emerges as a powerful solution, not only fostering physical stability but also promoting a myriad of health benefits.

As the body ages, the neuromuscular system changes, affecting proprioception and muscle strength. These changes can contribute to an increased risk of falls and injuries among seniors. However, engaging in targeted balance exercises can counteract these effects, improving stability and reducing the likelihood of accidents.

What does exercise do to the body, especially for individuals in their golden years? Physical activity, specifically balance exercises, stimulates the nervous system, enhancing coordination and fine-tuning reflexes. These exercises also strengthen the core muscles, essential for maintaining an upright posture and steadiness on one's feet. Additionally, they contribute to bone density and joint flexibility, addressing common concerns associated with aging, such as osteoporosis.

As we explore balance exercises for seniors, this isn't just about preventing falls. It's about empowering individuals to lead active, independent lives. From simple routines like

Standing on one leg to more dynamic exercises incorporating elements of strength and flexibility, a tailored approach can significantly enhance overall balance. This journey not only promotes physical well-being but also fosters mental resilience as individuals gain confidence in their movements and abilities.

In exploring balance exercises for those in their 60s and beyond, we delve into the significance of such activities and provide practical insights into incorporating them into daily routines. Embracing the transformative power of exercise, elders can navigate the aging process with grace, maintaining a sense of stability both in body and spirit.

Benefits of Exercise

- **Physical Health:** Regular exercise is crucial for maintaining optimal physical health. It improves general cardiovascular health, lowers the risk of chronic illnesses, including diabetes and heart disease, and aids with weight control.

- **Mental Well-being:** Exercise has a significant impact on mental well-being. It stimulates the production of endorphins, known as "feel-good" hormones. It can alleviate symptoms of depression and anxiety, promoting a positive mood.

- **Improved Sleep Quality:** Engaging in regular physical activity contributes to better sleep patterns. Quality sleep is essential for cognitive function, mood regulation, and well-being.

- **Enhanced Cognitive Function:** Exercise has been associated with improved cognitive performance and a decreased likelihood of mental deterioration with age. It boosts blood flow to the brain, supports the growth of new neurons, and enhances memory and learning.

- **Increased Energy Levels:** Contrary to the misconception that exercise depletes energy, it boosts energy levels. Regular physical activity improves muscle strength and endurance, making daily tasks easier and reducing feelings of fatigue.

- **Social Interaction:** Many forms of exercise involve social engagement, whether joining a sports team, attending fitness classes, or working out with friends. It fosters a sense of community and can positively impact mental well-being.

- **Stress Reduction:** Exercise is a natural stress reliever by reducing levels of the body's stress hormones, such as cortisol. It provides an outlet for pent-up tension and helps in maintaining emotional balance.

- **Enhanced Immune System:** Regular moderate-intensity exercise has been associated with a more robust immune system. It could improve the body's ability to fend against diseases and infections.

- **Increased Lifespan:** Numerous studies suggest that regular exercise increases longevity. The combination of physical and mental health benefits contributes to an overall healthier and longer life.

- **Weight Management:** Exercise, in combination with a balanced diet, is a critical factor in managing body weight. It helps burn calories and build muscle mass, supporting weight loss and maintenance.

Types of Exercise

- **Cardiovascular Exercises:** Cardio exercises focus on improving the health of the heart and circulatory system. Running, cycling, swimming, and brisk walking are a few examples. These activities increase heart rate, improve lung capacity, and enhance cardiovascular fitness.

- **Strength Training:** Strength training involves resistance exercises to build muscle mass and strength. Weight lifting, bodyweight exercises, and resistance band workouts fall under this category. It not only contributes to better muscle tone but also boosts metabolism and helps in weight management.

- **Flexibility Workouts:** Flexibility exercises aim to enhance joint mobility and reduce the risk of injuries. Some common kinds of flexibility training include yoga, Pilates, and stretching. These activities improve range of motion, balance, and posture.

- **Balance Training:** Balance exercises are crucial for stability and preventing falls, especially as individuals age. Activities such as stretches, stability ball exercises, and specific yoga poses help improve balance and coordination.

- **Interval Training:** Interval training alternates between short bursts of intense activity and periods of rest or lower-intensity exercise. This approach enhances both cardiovascular fitness and calorie burning. An increasingly common interval training type is High-Intensity Interval Training (HIIT).

- **Functional Fitness:** Functional workouts enhance regular activities by imitating real-life movements. These include squats, lunges, and movements that engage multiple muscle groups simultaneously. Functional fitness enhances overall strength and coordination.

- **Mind-Body Exercises:** Mind-body exercises focus on the connection between mental and physical well-being. Yoga and meditation fall into this category, promoting relaxation, stress reduction, and mindfulness.

- **Rehabilitative Exercises:** Targeted exercises help individuals recover from injuries or surgery. Physical therapy exercises, rehabilitation workouts, and specific movements prescribed by healthcare professionals aid recovery.

- **Outdoor Activities:** Engaging in outdoor activities such as hiking, trail running, or playing sports not only provides physical benefits but also offers the mental and emotional advantages of being in nature.

- **Cross-Training:** Cross-training involves incorporating various exercises into a routine to prevent monotony, reduce the risk of overuse injuries, and achieve overall fitness. It may include a combination of cardiovascular, strength, and flexibility workouts.

Chapter 1: Importance of Balance for Seniors

Maintaining balance is a crucial aspect of overall health, and for seniors, it takes on even greater significance. The aging process brings about natural changes in the body, such as decreased muscle mass, changes in vision, and reduced flexibility, all of which can contribute to a decline in balance.

One of the primary reasons balance is crucial for seniors is the prevention of falls. According to the Centers for Disease Control and Prevention (CDC), falls are a leading cause of injury among older adults, often resulting in fractures, head injuries, and a decline in overall well-being. By incorporating balance exercises into a senior's fitness routine, we can enhance their stability and reduce the risk of falls.

Improved balance also translates into increased independence. Seniors with better balance can confidently navigate their surroundings, perform daily activities, and maintain an active lifestyle. It not only contributes to their physical well-being but also boosts their mental and emotional health.

Balance training for seniors goes beyond preventing falls; it promotes better posture and body awareness. Strengthening the core muscles, including the abdomen and lower back, is pivotal in maintaining an upright posture and preventing slouching, which can lead to discomfort and pain.

Engaging in activities that challenge proprioception, the body's ability to sense its position in space, is another crucial aspect of balance training for seniors. It can include exercises like standing on one leg, heel-to-toe walks, or incorporating stability balls into workouts. By continually challenging and improving proprioception, seniors can enhance their coordination and reaction time.

Benefits of Regular Balance Exercise

- **Improved Stability:** Regular balance exercises for seniors help enhance stability by targeting muscles and joints that maintain an upright posture. It reduces the risk of falls and related injuries.

- **Enhanced Coordination:** Balance exercises promote better coordination between muscle groups and sensory systems. It is particularly beneficial for seniors as it helps them navigate daily activities more quickly and confidently.

- **Fall Prevention:** One of the primary benefits of regular balance exercises is the significant reduction in the risk of falls. More robust balance and stability contribute to a more secure footing, reducing the likelihood of accidents and injuries.

- **Increased Flexibility:** Balance exercises often involve a range of motion, which helps improve flexibility in joints and muscles. This increased flexibility contributes to better overall mobility and reduces stiffness associated with aging.

- **Muscle Strengthening:** Balancing requires the activation of various muscle groups, leading to improved strength. It is crucial for seniors as it aids in maintaining muscle mass, which tends to decline with age, and supports overall physical function.

- **Enhanced Posture:** Good balance is closely tied to proper posture. Regular balance exercises help seniors develop and maintain better posture, which not only contributes to physical well-being but also positively impacts confidence and self-esteem.

- **Cognitive Benefits:** Balance exercises often involve focus and concentration, which can contribute to cognitive health. Seniors engaging in these exercises may experience improved mental alertness and sharper cognitive function.

- **Joint Health:** The controlled movements in balance exercises promote joint health by facilitating fluid motion and reducing stiffness. It is essential for seniors dealing with conditions like arthritis.

- **Independence:** Ultimately, the culmination of these benefits leads to increased independence for seniors. Better balance and stability empower them to perform daily tasks more confidently, maintaining a higher quality of life.

Science Behind Balance for Seniors

- **Vestibular System:** The inner ear's vestibular system plays a crucial role in maintaining balance for seniors. This system detects changes in head movement and helps the brain understand the body's position in space.

- **Visual Input:** Vision is a significant contributor to balance. As seniors age, changes in vision, such as reduced depth perception and peripheral vision, can impact their ability to maintain balance. Regular eye check-ups and corrective lenses are essential.

- **Muscle Strength and Tone:** Maintaining solid and toned muscles is vital for balance in seniors. Regular strength training exercises, focusing on the core, legs, and lower body, can help enhance stability and reduce the risk of falls.

- **Joint Flexibility:** Flexible joints contribute to better balance and coordination. Stretching exercises aimed at improving joint flexibility, especially in the ankles, knees, and hips, can be beneficial for seniors.

- **Proprioception:** The body's ability to sense its position in space without relying on vision. Proprioception diminishes with age, but targeted exercises, such as standing on one leg or incorporating balance exercises into daily activities, can help improve proprioceptive abilities.

- **Neurological Health:** A healthy nervous system is crucial for maintaining balance. Regular physical activity and mental stimulation can contribute to overall neurological health, reducing the risk of falls.

- **Foot Health:** Proper footwear and foot care are often overlooked but are crucial for balance. Seniors should wear well-fitted shoes with nonskid soles to reduce the risk of slipping and falling.

- **Medication Management:** Some medications can have side effects that affect balance. Seniors should regularly review their medicines with healthcare professionals to ensure they are not contributing to balance issues.

- **Hydration and Nutrition:** Dehydration and poor nutrition can impact overall health, including balance. Seniors should maintain proper hydration and a well-balanced diet to support their physical well-being.

- **Regular Assessments:** Periodic assessments by healthcare professionals, including balance assessments, can help identify issues early on and tailor interventions to maintain or improve seniors' balance.

Chapter 2: Understanding Balance

How Balance Changes with Age

As individuals progress through the stages of life, the concept of balance undergoes a transformative journey, particularly for seniors. Balance, a crucial aspect of physical well-being, tends to change significantly with age, presenting unique challenges and considerations for older people.

One of the primary factors influencing balance in seniors is the natural aging process. As people age, there is a gradual decline in muscle mass, strength, and flexibility. This physiological shift can impact the body's ability to maintain equilibrium, making seniors more susceptible to falls and accidents. The decline in joint flexibility and the weakening of muscles can compromise stability, leading to an increased risk of stumbling or losing balance.

Moreover, sensory changes are pivotal in how balance evolves with age. Vision, proprioception (the body's awareness of its position in space), and the vestibular system (responsible for balance and spatial orientation) all experience age-related changes. Diminished vision, for example, may affect depth perception and make it challenging for seniors to navigate their surroundings safely. Changes in proprioception and the vestibular system can further contribute to instability.

Chronic health conditions and medications commonly associated with aging can exacerbate balance issues. Conditions such as arthritis, osteoporosis, and neurological disorders can impact the musculoskeletal system, hindering mobility and stability. Additionally, certain medications may have side effects such as dizziness or lightheadedness, further complicating the maintenance of balance.

To address these age-related balance changes, seniors can benefit from regular exercise programs focusing on strength, flexibility, and balance training. Activities like tai chi and yoga have been shown to enhance stability and reduce the risk of falls. Home modifications and assistive devices can also create safer environments for seniors.

Understanding these changes and implementing appropriate strategies can contribute to maintaining a higher quality of life and minimizing the risks associated with impaired balance in the elderly population.

Causes of Balance Loss in Seniors

- **Age-related Changes:** As individuals age, various physiological changes occur in the body, including a decline in muscle mass, joint flexibility, and bone density. These changes can affect posture and stability, making seniors more prone to balance issues.

- **Inner Ear Disorders:** The inner ear plays a crucial role in maintaining balance by providing information about the body's position in space. Disorders such as

Meniere's disease or vestibular neuritis can affect the inner ear, leading to dizziness and imbalance.

- **Neurological Conditions:** Conditions like Parkinson's disease, stroke, or neuropathy can affect the nervous system, compromising signals between the brain and muscles responsible for maintaining balance.

- **Medication Side Effects:** Certain medications prescribed for other health conditions may have side effects that impact balance. Seniors should be aware of the potential effects of their drugs and discuss any concerns with their healthcare providers.

- **Muscle Weakness and Joint Problems:** Weakness in the muscles, particularly those in the lower body, and joint issues such as arthritis can contribute to instability and difficulty maintaining balance.

- **Vision Impairment:** Diminished visual acuity or eye conditions like cataracts can affect a senior's ability to perceive their surroundings accurately, increasing the risk of falls.

- **Dehydration:** Inadequate fluid intake can lead to dehydration, affecting blood pressure and causing dizziness or lightheadedness, contributing to balance problems.

- **Lack of Physical Activity:** Sedentary lifestyles can weaken muscles and reduce flexibility, making it more challenging for seniors to maintain balance.

Symptoms of Balance Loss in Seniors:

- **Dizziness or Lightheadedness:** Feeling dizzy or lightheaded, especially when standing up, can be an early indicator of balance issues.

- **Frequent Falls:** Seniors experiencing balance problems are more prone to falls, resulting in injuries and a fear of falling, further limiting their mobility.

- **Difficulty Walking:** An unsteady gait or difficulty walking in a straight line may indicate compromised balance.

- **Vertigo:** Sensations of spinning or a spinning environment, known as vertigo, may be associated with inner ear disorders affecting balance.

- **Muscle Weakness:** Weakness in the legs and difficulty rising from a seated position may contribute to balance challenges.

- **Changes in Posture:** Seniors with balance issues may exhibit changes in posture, such as leaning forward or to the side, to maintain stability.

- **Decline in Coordination:** Reduced coordination and difficulty with tasks that require precise movements may be signs of balance impairment.

Factors Affecting Balance in Seniors

Maintaining balance is a crucial aspect of overall well-being, especially for seniors who may face increased challenges due to age-related body changes. Several factors contribute to the delicate equilibrium for stable mobility in older individuals.

One primary factor is age-related changes in the sensory systems, particularly vision and proprioception. As individuals age, there is a natural decline in visual acuity and depth perception, making it more challenging to perceive and navigate the environment accurately. Similarly, proprioception, the body's ability to sense its position in space, may diminish, affecting balance and coordination.

Muscle strength and flexibility also play pivotal roles in maintaining balance. Seniors often experience a gradual loss of muscle mass and strength, leading to reduced stability. Weakness in the lower body, especially the legs and core muscles, can compromise an individual's ability to support themselves and respond effectively to changes in posture.

Neurological changes, including a decline in reaction time and processing speed, contribute to diminished balance in seniors. The brain's ability to receive and interpret signals from the sensory organs and subsequently generate appropriate motor responses may slow down with age, impacting the speed and efficiency of balance-related actions.

Chronic health conditions and medication side effects are additional factors influencing balance in seniors. Conditions such as arthritis, osteoporosis, and inner ear disorders can directly affect stability. Furthermore, certain medications may induce dizziness or lightheadedness, increasing the risk of falls.

Environmental factors, such as uneven surfaces, poor lighting, and inadequate footwear, can pose significant challenges to seniors. A lack of proper home modifications or assistive devices may increase the risk of falls and injuries.

Seated Leg Lifts

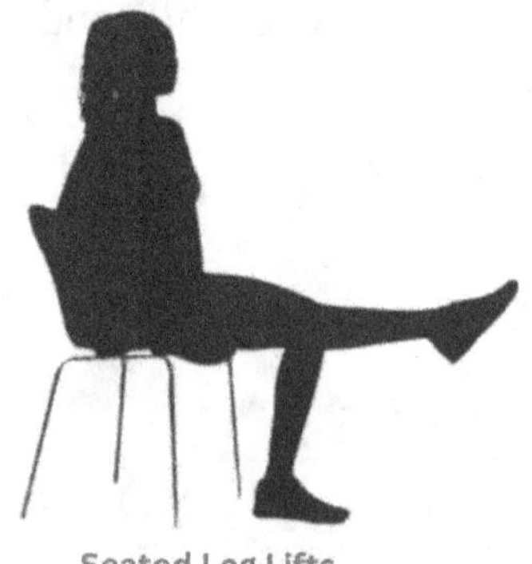

Seated Leg Lifts

- Sit on a sturdy chair with a straight back and feet flat on the floor.

- Place your hands on the sides of the chair for support and stability.

- Inhale, engage your core and lift one leg straight before you.

- Keep the lifted leg straight and parallel to the ground without locking your knee.

- Exhale as you lower the leg, stopping just before it touches the floor.

- Repeat on the other leg, alternating in a controlled and deliberate motion.

- Aim for 10-15 repetitions on each leg, gradually increasing as your strength improves.

- This exercise targets the core, thighs, and hip flexors, promoting strength and flexibility.

Seated Knee-to-Chest

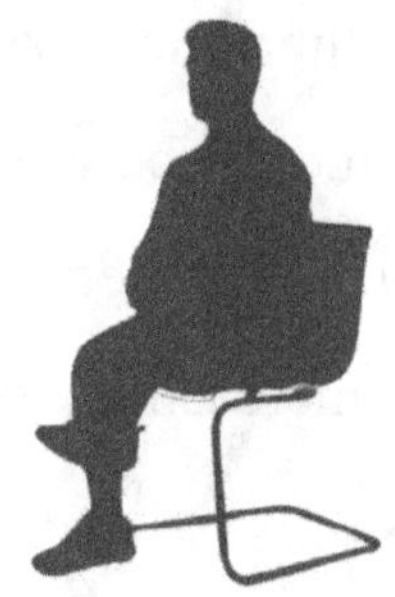

Seated Knee-to-Chest

- Sit on a chair with your legs extended in front of you.
- One leg should be bent and brought to your chest.
- Hold the shin or knee with both hands, maintaining a straight back.
- Gently pull the knee closer to your chest, feeling a stretch in your lower back and hip.

- Hold the stretch for 15-30 seconds, breathing deeply.
- Release and switch to the other leg.
- Repeat the sequence for a balanced stretch.

Seated Backbend

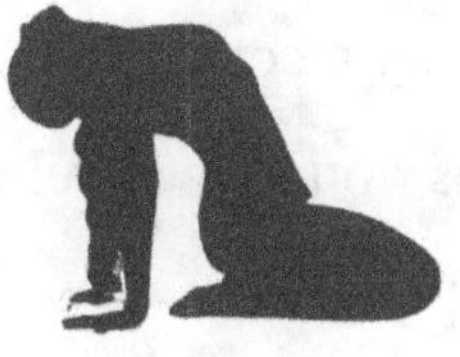

Seated Backbend

- Kneel on the mat with your legs extended at the back.

- Put your hands behind your back with your fingers pointing in that direction.
- Inhale deeply, lengthening your spine, and lift your chest toward the ceiling.
- Arch your back, gently dropping your head backward.
- Keep your shoulders relaxed, engaging your core for stability.
- Feel a stretch in your chest, shoulders, and front of the hips.
- Hold the position for a few breaths, maintaining a comfortable stretch.
- Exhale as you slowly release, returning to a seated position.
- This seated backbend improves flexibility, opens the chest, and energizes the spine.

Toe Raises

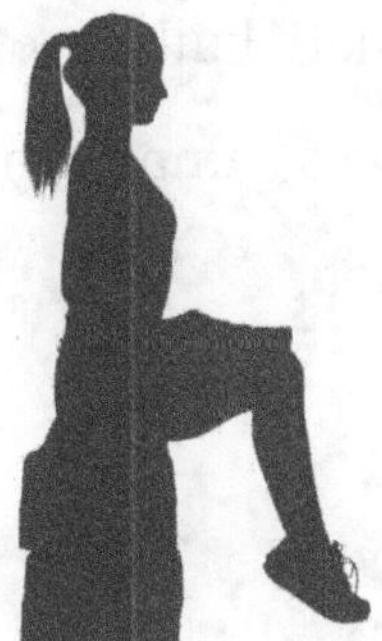

Toe Raises

- Sit with your feet hip-width apart, ensuring good posture with shoulders back and core engaged.
- Lift your heels off the ground by pushing through the balls of your feet, rising as high as possible.
- To activate the calf muscles, maintain the elevated posture briefly.
- With steady movement, return your heels to the floor.

- Perform three sets of 15-20 repetitions for an effective calf-strengthening workout.
- Toe raises help build strength and stability in the calves, improving overall lower body function.

Seated Trunk Circles

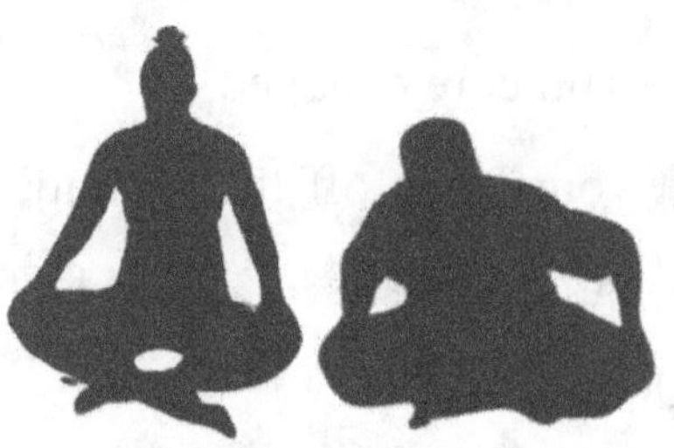

Seated Trunk Circles

- Sit on the mat with legs folded, elongating the spine.

- Keep the spine straight and shoulders relaxed.
- Place your hands on your knee to stabilize your upper body.
- Start circling your torso in a clockwise direction. Move your shoulders, chest, and hips in a smooth, circular motion.
- Perform controlled and deliberate movements to avoid straining your back or neck. Focus on engaging your core muscles.
- Maintain a steady breathing pattern throughout the exercise. Inhale as you rotate backward, and exhale as you rotate forward.
- Aim for a full range of motion without forcing any movement. Gradually increase

the size of your circles as your flexibility improves.

- After completing several circles in one direction, switch to counterclockwise rotations. This rotation helps balance the workout and targets different muscles.

- Perform 10-15 repetitions in each direction, or adjust based on your fitness level. Once you feel more at ease with the workout, increase the number.

- Trunk circles work well as a warm-up before more intense exercises, promoting flexibility and loosening your core muscles.

Seated Marching

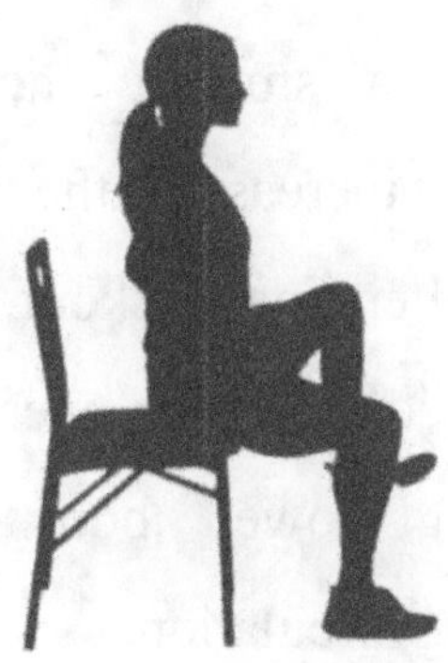

Seated Marching

- Sit upright on a sturdy chair with feet flat on the floor and knees bent at a 90-degree angle.

- Lift one knee toward the chest while keeping the back straight and shoulders relaxed.

- Lower the lifted knee and repeat the movement with the other leg.

- Continue alternating legs in a controlled marching motion.

- Engage the core muscles throughout the exercise to enhance stability and balance.

- Aim for a smooth and steady pace, gradually increasing the intensity for a more challenging workout.

- This seated marching exercise is ideal for improving lower body strength and promoting circulation.

Seated Forward Punch

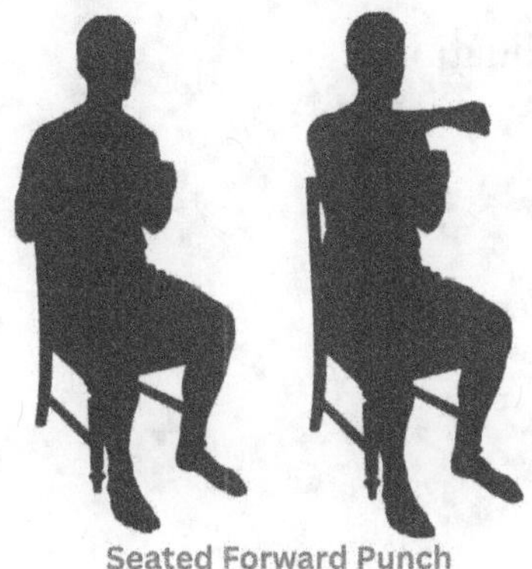

Seated Forward Punch

- Sit upright with both feet placed firmly on the ground.

- Extend your right arm into a powerful punch.

- Visualize punching through an imaginary barrier in front of you, maximizing the extension of your arm.

- Perform for 30-45 seconds, retract your arm, and step back to the starting position.

- This exercise strengthens the core, legs, and arms and enhances balance and coordination.

Hip Flexion Fold

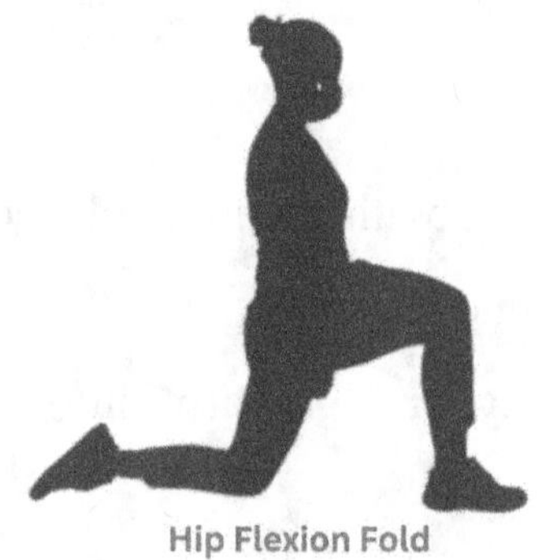

Hip Flexion Fold

- Begin by kneeling on your left leg, ensuring your right leg is bent in front at a 90-degree angle.
- Gradually shift your weight forward, emphasizing a gentle lean into the stretch.

- Maintain the stretched position for about 15-30 seconds, feeling the tension ease.

- Transition to kneeling on your right leg and repeat the exercise with your left leg bent.

- This exercise enhances hip flexibility, reduces tightness in the hip flexors, and promotes lower body mobility.

Seated Hip Stretch

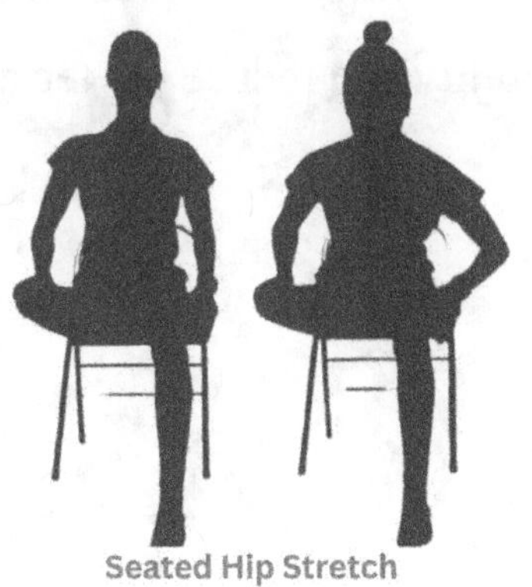

Seated Hip Stretch

- Sit on the chair with your legs planted firmly on the floor.
- Bend your right knee and place the sole of your right foot on the thigh of your left leg.
- Keep your back straight and gently hinge forward from your hips.
- Hold the stretch for 15-30 seconds, feeling the stretch in your right hip and buttock.
- Repeat the stretch on the other side after switching legs.
- Perform 2-3 sets on each side to improve flexibility and reduce hip tension.

Seated Overhead Stretch

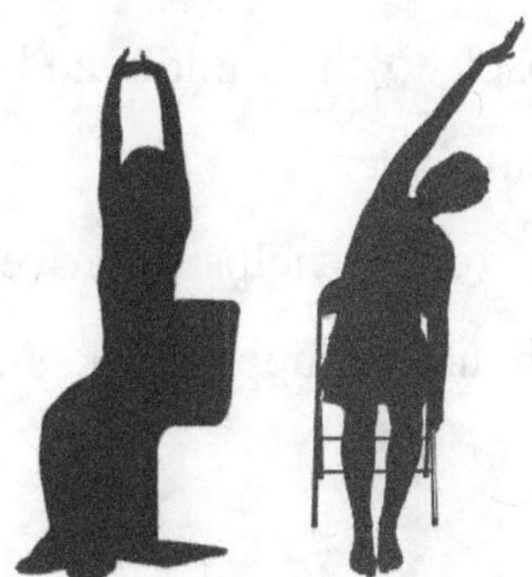

Seated Overhead Stretch

- Sit comfortably on the floor with your legs crossed or in a chair with your feet flat on the ground.
- Extend your arms overhead, clasping your hands together.
- Inhale deeply and lengthen your spine.
- As you exhale, gently lean to one side, feeling a stretch along the opposite side of your torso.

- Hold the stretch for 15-30 seconds, breathing deeply.
- Go back to the middle and repeat on the opposite side.
- This exercise helps improve flexibility in the shoulders, upper back, and sides of the body.

Chapter 4: Standing Exercise

Tree Pose

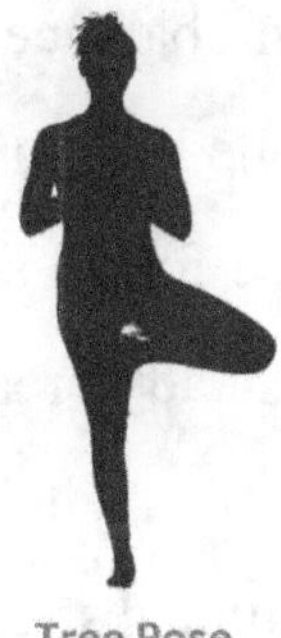

Tree Pose

- Stand tall with your feet together, weight evenly distributed.
- Shift your weight to your left foot and lift your right foot, placing the sole against the inner thigh or calf.

- Find your balance, engage your core, and bring your palms together in a prayer session.

- Inhale deeply, extending your arms overhead with your fingers reaching toward the sky.

- To maintain balance, keep your eyes focused on one location.

- Hold the pose for 30 seconds to a minute, focusing on steady breath.

- Slowly release, switch sides, and repeat for a well-rounded stretch.

- Tree Pose strengthens legs, improves balance, and promotes mental focus.

Flamingo Stand

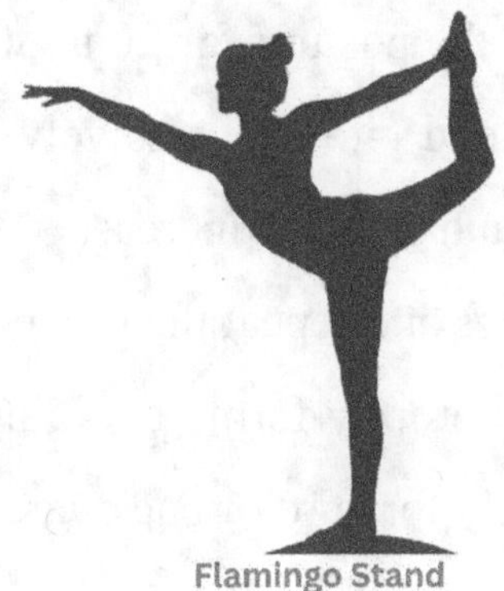

Flamingo Stand

- Begin by standing on one leg with your feet hip-width apart.

- Lift your opposite leg off the ground, bending at the knee.

- Extend the lifted leg backward, engaging core muscles.

- Bring your torso forward, keeping your back straight, and extend one arm in front for balance, and use them to hold the lifted leg.

- Engage your core for stability and focus on a fixed point to help balance.

- Maintain the posture for 20 to 30 seconds, then extend it progressively as your strength and stability increase.

- Switch legs and repeat the process.

- Maintain proper form, avoiding leaning excessively forward or backward.

- Incorporate this exercise into your routine for improved balance, core strength, and flexibility.

Arm Raises

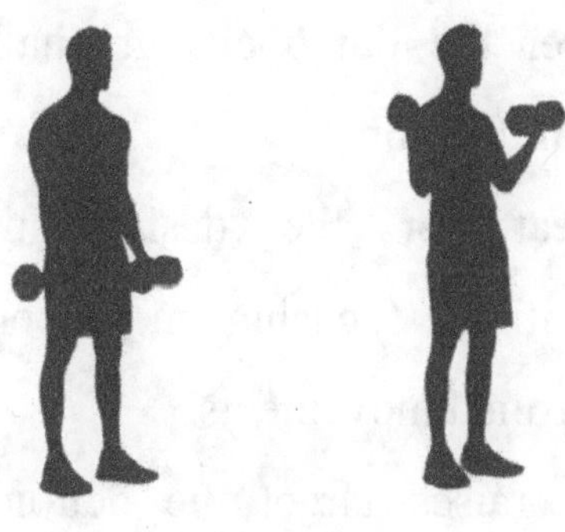

Arm Raises

- Maintain a straight back and a tight core while standing with your feet shoulder-width apart.

- Hold a dumbbell in each hand, palms facing your body, and arms extended down by your sides.

- In a controlled motion, lift both arms simultaneously to shoulder height, maintaining a slight bend in your elbows.

- Pause at the top of the movement, squeezing your shoulder muscles.

- Lower the dumbbells gradually to their initial position.

- Repeat for the desired number of repetitions, focusing on proper form and controlled movements.

- Arm raises target the deltoid muscles, helping to strengthen and tone your shoulders.

Wood Chop

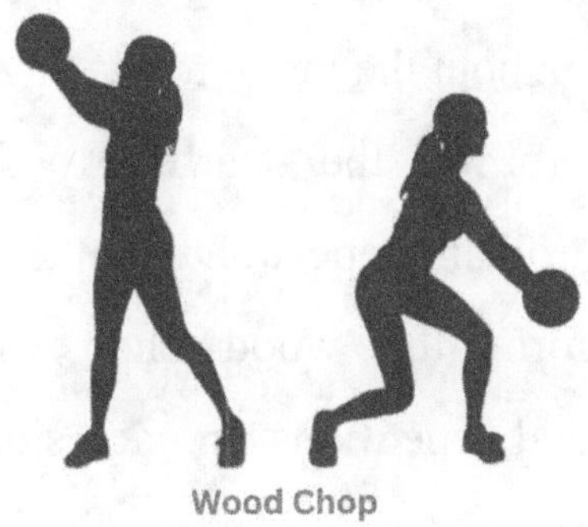

Wood Chop

- Stand with feet shoulder-width apart, holding a single dumbbell or medicine ball with both hands.

- Begin with the weight at one side of your body, arms extended.

- Engage your core and twist your torso, bringing the weight diagonally across your body and above the opposite shoulder.

- Pivot your back foot and bend your knees slightly as you rotate.

- Keep your arms straight and controlled throughout the movement.

- Return to the starting position with control, and repeat on the other side.

- Perform the wood chop exercise for several repetitions on each side, focusing on proper form and controlled movement.

Squats

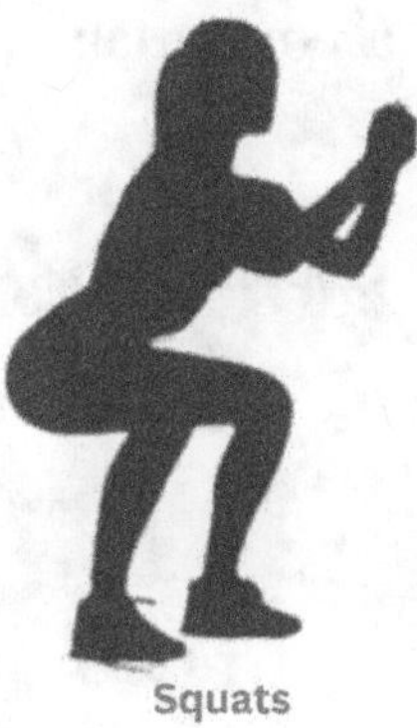

Squats

- Stand with your feet tall and apart.

- Keep your chest up and shoulders back.

- Begin by bending your knees and pushing your hips back.

- Lower your body as if you are sitting back in a chair.

- Lower yourself till your thighs are in line with the floor.

- Keep your knees in line with your toes, not extending past them.

- Put some pressure on your heels to get back to your starting position.
- Start with a comfortable number of 8-12 repetitions.
- Gradually increase as your strength improves.

Heel Raises

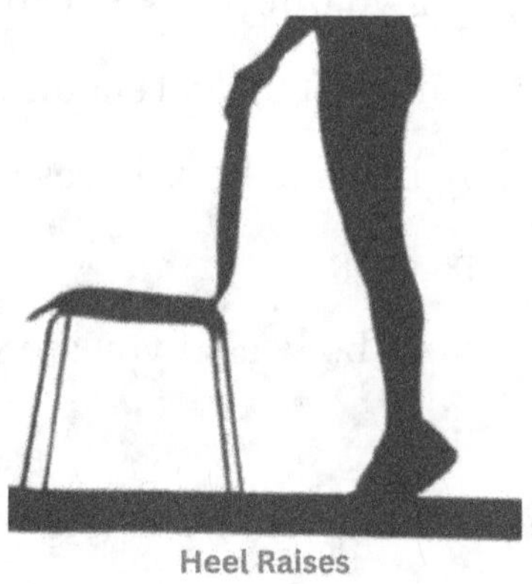

Heel Raises

- Maintain proper posture by keeping your shoulders back and your core tight while standing with your feet hip-width apart.

- Elevate your heels off the ground and ascend onto your toes.

- Place a chair in front of you, holding it as a support.

- Hold the raised position momentarily, feeling the contraction in your calf muscles.

- Lower your heels back down to the ground slowly and with control.

- Repeat the motion for several repetitions, gradually increasing as your strength improves.

- This exercise strengthens your calves, improves ankle stability, and promotes lower leg fitness.

Mini Lunges

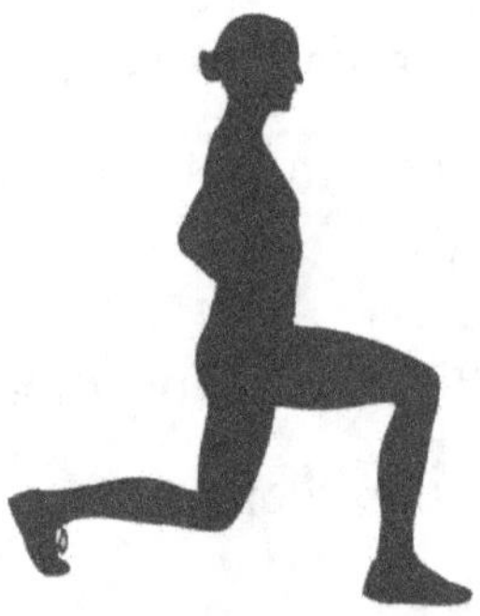

- Stand with feet hip-width apart and engage your core muscles.

- Maintaining an upright posture, take a stride forward with your right foot.

- Bend both of your knees to a 90-degree angle to lower your torso.

- Ensure your front knee is directly above your ankle and your back knee hovers above the ground.

- Go back to the beginning position by pushing through your right heel.

- Using a different leg for each repetition, repeat on the other.

- Aim for two sets of 12-15 repetitions on each leg.

- Focus on controlled movements to target your quads, hamstrings, and glutes.

3-Way Hip Kick

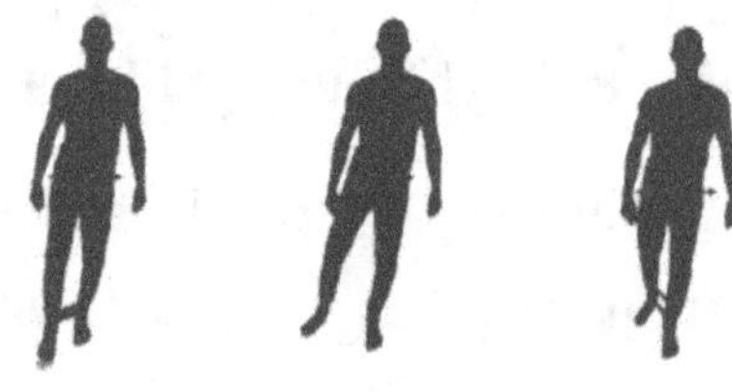

3-Way Hip Kick

- Begin by standing upright with a resistance band looped lightly around your ankles.
- Ensure a level pelvis as you kick one-foot length in front.
- Maintain balance on the opposite foot throughout the movement.
- Extend the foot sideways after the forward kick.

- Maintain pelvis stability as you kick one-foot length behind you.
- Emphasize straight legs throughout the backward movement.
- Aim to perform sets without letting the foot touch the ground between kicks.
- Repeat the sequence 5-10 times for each leg.

Wall Push-ups

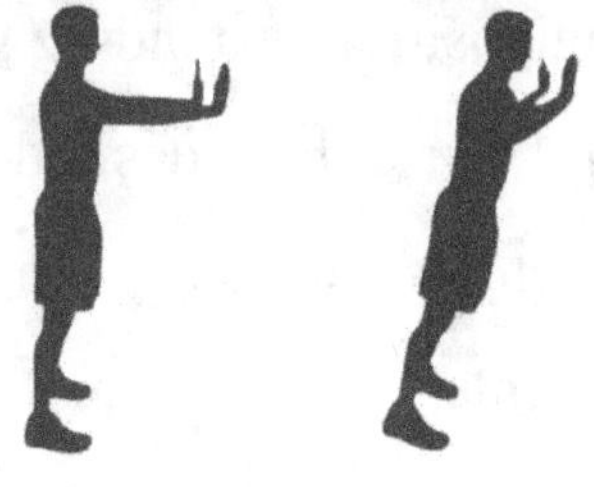

Wall Push-ups

- Stand facing a wall with your feet hip-width apart.
- With your hands slightly wider than shoulder-width apart, place them on the wall at shoulder height.
- Maintain a neutral spine, contract your core, and keep your body erect.
- Lower your chest toward the wall by bending your elbows while keeping your body straight.
- Inhale as you lower your chest towards the wall.
- Exhale as you push yourself back to the starting position, extending your arms.
- Repeat for the desired number of repetitions, focusing on controlled movements.

Single Leg Stands

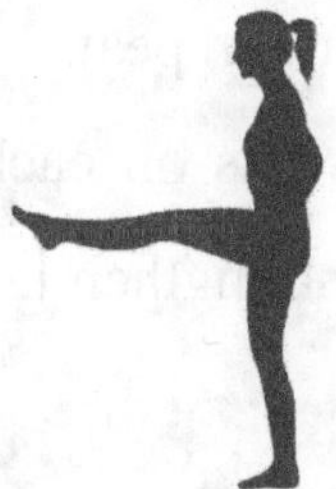

Single Leg Stands

- Start by standing with feet hip-width apart.

- Lift one foot and use the other leg to maintain balance.

- Keep the lifted leg slightly bent or extend it forward for more challenge.

- To stay stable, keep your back straight by using your core.

- To aid in balance, fix your attention on a particular spot.

- Hold the position for 15-30 seconds, gradually increasing as you get comfortable.
- Switch legs and repeat.
- Perform 2-3 sets on each leg to improve balance and strengthen leg muscles.

Chapter 5: Walking Exercises

Lateral Step

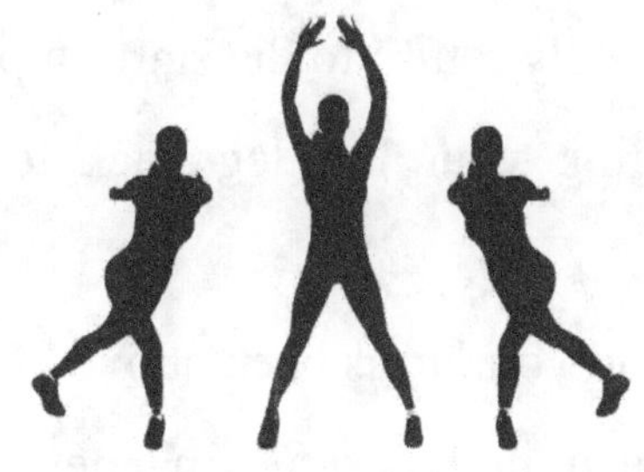

Lateral Step

- Start by placing your feet a little wider apart than shoulder-width apart.
- Extend both hands above your head, keeping a straight posture.
- Initiate the exercise by taking a substantial step back with your left leg.

- Cross the left leg diagonally behind the right leg.

- Bend the front knee (right) as you pull your arms back towards your sides.

- Engage your core for stability.

- Gradually return to the starting position by bringing your left leg back to meet the right.

- Extend your arms back above your head.

- Proceed in the same manner across the other side.

Walking Lunge

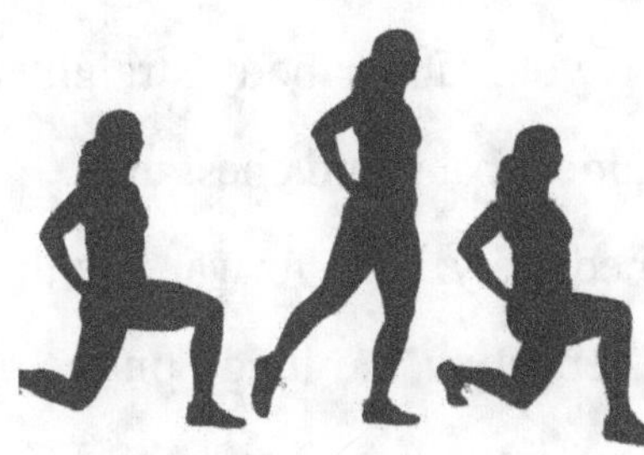

Walking Lunge

- Stand with feet hip-width apart and hands on hips or by your sides.

- Take a controlled step forward with your right leg, ensuring the weight is on your heel.

- Bend the right knee, lowering your body until your right thigh is parallel to the floor, keeping the rear knee slightly above the ground. Aim for a 90-degree angle in the right knee and hip.

- Bring your left foot forward, tapping it to the floor or hovering it for a more advanced variation.

- Keep your upper body straight with your shoulders back and chest up

- Immediately step forward with your left leg, repeating the lunge on the other side. Ensure both knees and the left hip form 90-degree angles.

- With each stride, continue to walk in a lunge, switching your legs.

Walking Knee Hugs

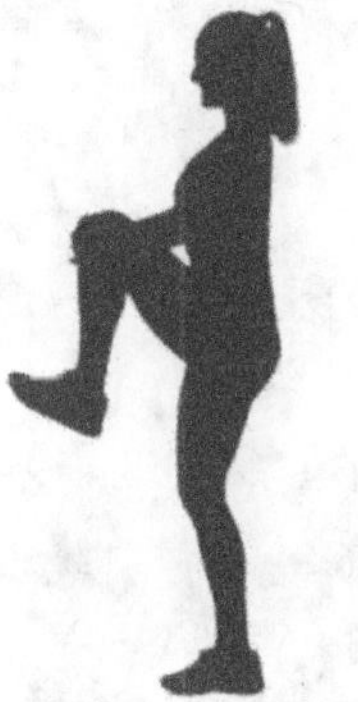

Walking Knee Hugs

- Stand tall with feet hip-width apart.

- Engage core muscles for stability.

- Lift right knee towards the chest, holding with both hands.

- Hug right knee to chest, feeling a stretch in your hip flexors.

- Keep back straight and shoulders relaxed.

- Release the right leg, and take a step forward.

- Repeat with left knee, alternating legs.

- Perform at a controlled pace.

- Aim for 10-15 reps on each leg.

Heel-to-Toe Walk

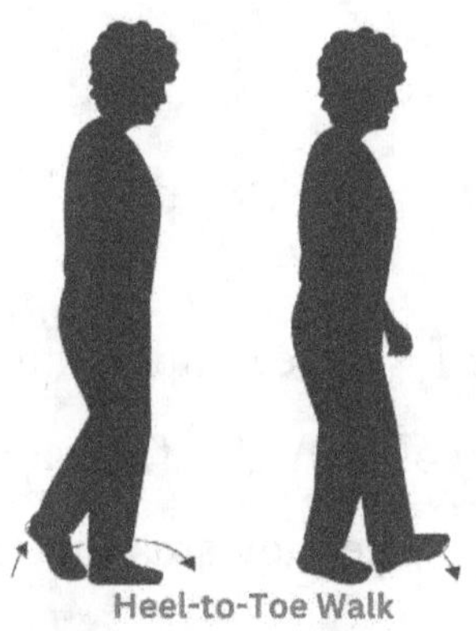

Heel-to-Toe Walk

- Step your feet together and maintain a sideways posture with your arms.

- Lift your right heel off the ground, keeping your toes in contact with the floor.

- Place your right heel before your left toes, ensuring they touch or overlap.

- Shift your body weight onto the right foot.

- Lift your left heel, bring it in front, and place it in line with or slightly overlapping your right toes.

- Alternate heel-to-toe steps, maintaining a straight line and focusing on balance.

- For added stability, extend your arms to the sides or in front of you.

- Keep your gaze straight ahead to help maintain balance.

- Perform the exercise slowly and with control, emphasizing balance over speed.

Marching on the Spot with Arms

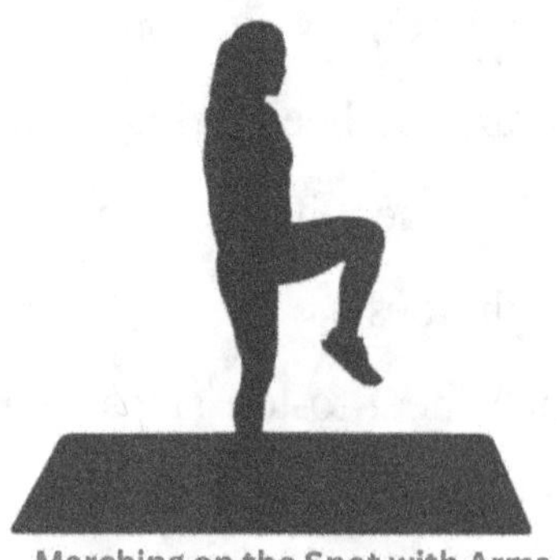

Marching on the Spot with Arms

- Stand with feet shoulder-width apart.
- Lift knees alternately while keeping arms bent at a 90-degree angle.
- Engage core muscles and maintain a brisk, steady pace.
- Ensure proper posture with shoulders relaxed and back straight.
- Continue marching for a set duration or number of reps.

- Increase intensity by incorporating high knees or adding light weights.
- Focus on controlled movements for a full-body workout.

Walking Knee Ups

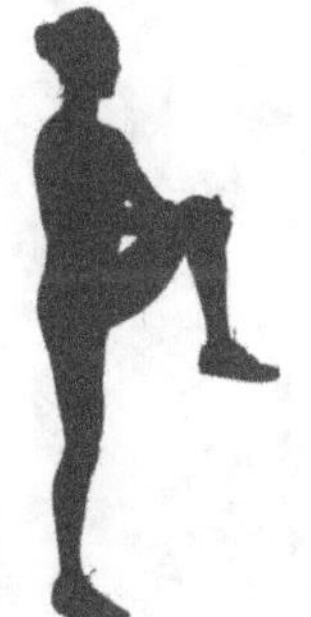

Walking Knee Ups

- Stand upright with feet shoulder-width apart.
- Lift your right knee towards your chest, keeping your core engaged.

- As you lower the right knee, lift the left knee in a fluid, alternating motion.

- Continue walking in place, bringing each knee up towards your chest.

- Maintain a brisk pace for an effective cardio and core workout.

- Aim for 15-20 repetitions on each leg, gradually increasing as your fitness improves.

Backward Walking

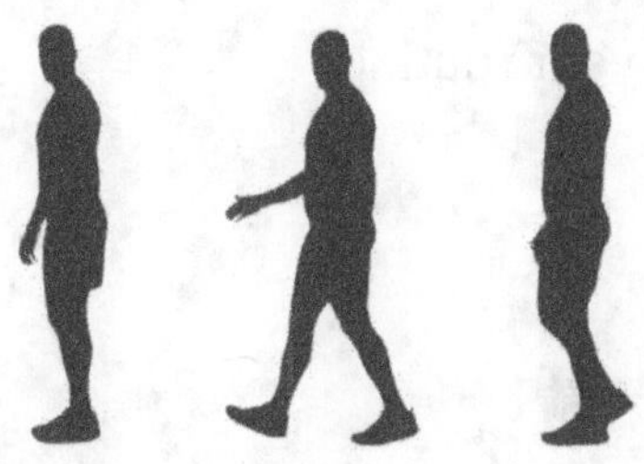

Backward Walking

- Stand with feet hip-width apart.
- Engage core muscles for stability.
- Move your right foot backward and take a step.
- Transfer weight to the right foot.
- Bring the left and right feet together.
- Repeat the backward steps, alternating legs.
- Focus on a smooth, controlled motion.

- Gradually increase the pace as comfort allows.
- Perform for 5-10 minutes, incorporating it into your routine.

Lateral Lunge

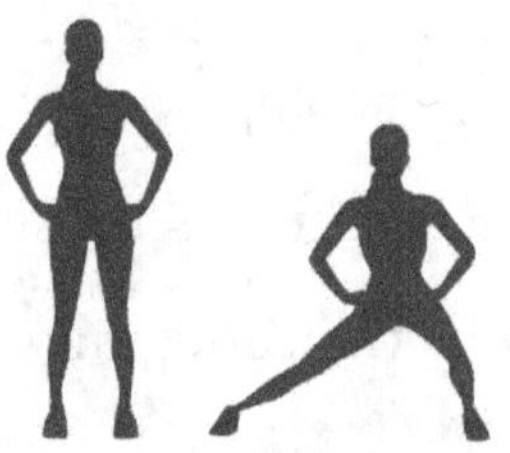

Lateral Lunge

- Stand with feet hip-width apart.
- Step to the side with your right foot, keeping your toes forward.

- Shift your body weight to the right, bending the right knee while keeping the left leg straight.

- Lower your body towards the right, keeping your back straight.

- Push through your right heel to get back to where you were.

- Repeat on the other side, alternating lunges.

Brisk Walking

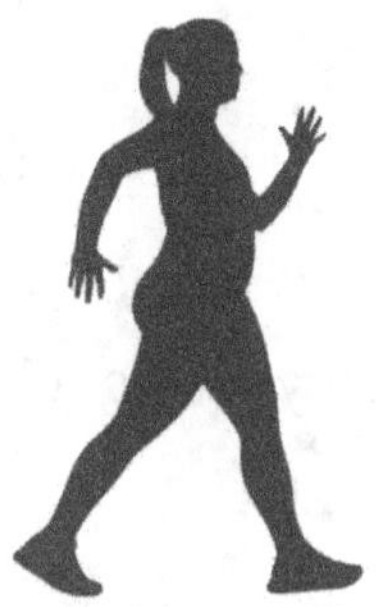

Brisk Walking

- Place your feet shoulder-width apart and stand upright.

- Keep your spine neutral and contract your core muscles.

- Swing your arms naturally as you start walking briskly.

- Take purposeful steps, landing on your heel and pushing off from your toes.

- Keep a brisk pace, aiming for 15-30 minutes of continuous walking.

- Maintain good posture throughout the exercise.

- Breathe deeply and rhythmically as you walk.

- Gradually increase speed or duration as your fitness improves.

Sideways Walking

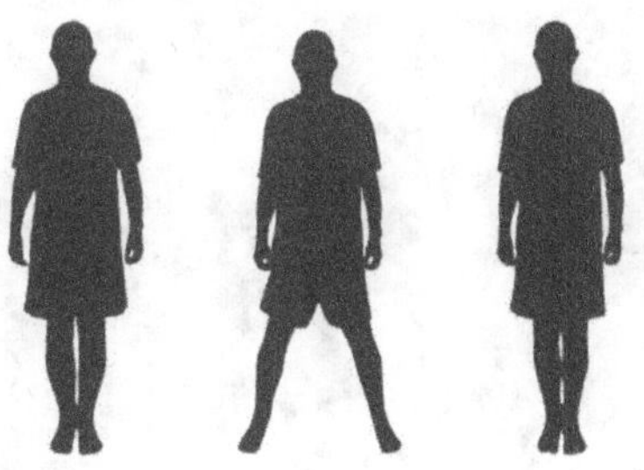

Sideways Walking

- Stand with your feet together, ensuring a slight knee bend for flexibility.

- Execute a deliberate and controlled sideways step, leading with one foot.
- Follow through by bringing the other foot to meet the lead foot.
- Maintain stable hips, avoiding any sagging during each step.
- Aim for ten steps in each direction or cover the entire width of the room with each purposeful lateral movement.

Chapter 6: Vestibular Exercise

Turning Side-to-Side

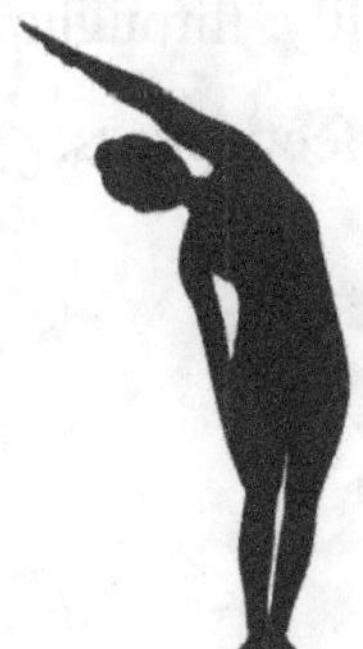

Turning Side-to-Side

- Stand with feet shoulder-width apart.
- Keep your core engaged, raise your left arm overhead, and keep your right arm at the side of your body.
- Slowly turn your upper body to the right.
- Hold for a moment, feeling the stretch in your torso.

- Return to the center and repeat the motion to the left.
- Perform 10-15 reps on each side, maintaining controlled movements.
- Breathe steadily throughout the exercise for optimal effectiveness.

Head Exercise

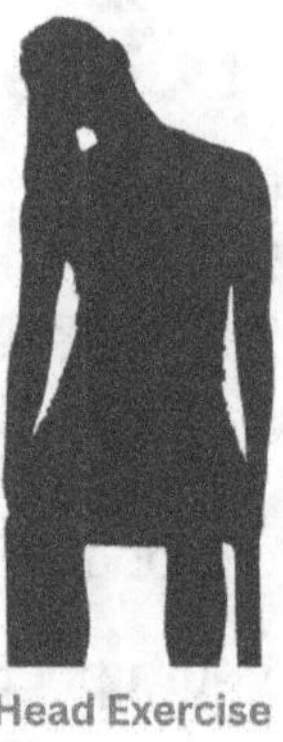

Head Exercise

- Sit or stand comfortably with a straight posture.

- Inhale deeply, and as you exhale, gently lower your chin to your chest, feeling a stretch in the back of your neck.
- Slowly roll your head to the right, bringing your ear towards your shoulder, and hold for a few seconds.
- Continue rolling your head back, looking up at the ceiling, and hold the stretch.
- Repeat the same motion to the left side.
- Gradually rotate your head in a circular motion, clockwise and then counterclockwise.
- Perform each movement slowly and with control, avoiding sudden or jerky motions.
- Repeat the entire sequence a few times to promote flexibility and reduce tension.

Shoulder Turns

- Stand with your feet shoulder-width apart.

- Keep your core engaged and maintain a straight posture.

- Slowly rotate your shoulders to the right, leading with your torso.

- Hold the position briefly, feeling the stretch in your upper back.

- Return to the starting position and repeat the rotation to the left.

- Perform 10-15 repetitions on each side, gradually increasing as you get comfortable.

- Breathe consistently throughout the exercise to enhance flexibility and range of motion.

Gaze Stabilization

- Sit comfortably: Find a quiet place to sit with good posture, either in a chair or on the floor.
- Choose a fixed point before you, like a dot on the wall or a small object.
- While keeping your head still, shift your gaze to the chosen point without moving your head.
- Maintain your focus on the point for about 30 seconds, trying to minimize head movement.
- After 30 seconds, slowly move your head from side to side or up and down, but keep your eyes on the same point.

- Repeat the exercise 5 times, gradually increasing the duration as your gaze stability improves.

Eye Movement: Up and Down

- Sit comfortably with your back straight and shoulders relaxed.
- Focus on a stationary point directly in front of you at eye level.
- Inhale deeply, then exhale slowly.
- Without moving your head, look upward as far as comfortable, then downward.
- Repeat this eye movement up and down for 10-15 repetitions.
- Blink a few times to relax your eyes.

- Take a brief break and repeat the exercise if desired.

Marching Hip Raises

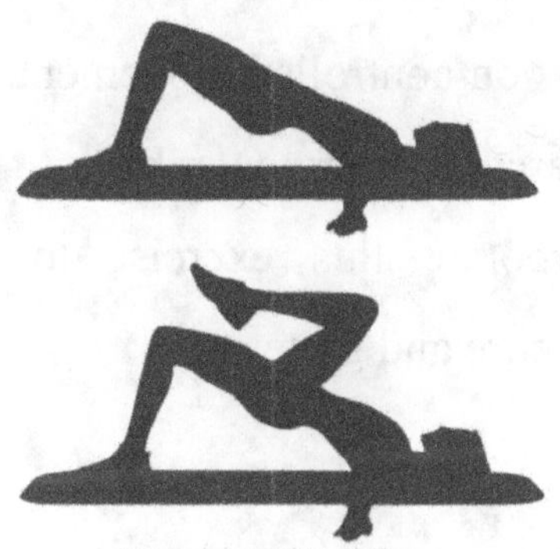

Marching Hip Raises

- Start by lying on your back with your knees bent and feet flat on the floor.
- Place your hands by your sides for stability.
- Lift your hips towards the ceiling, forming a straight line from shoulders to knees.

- Maintain the bridge position and march by lifting one knee towards your chest.

- Alternate legs in a controlled manner, keeping your core engaged.

- Repeat the marching motion for a set duration or number of reps.

- Focus on controlled movements and avoid overarching your lower back.

- Incorporate this exercise to strengthen your core and glutes.

Scissor Legs

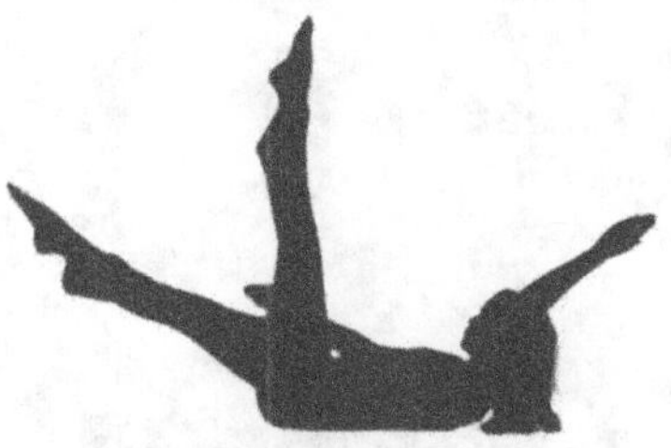

Scissor Legs

- Lie on your back with your hands under your hips for support.

- Lift your legs off the ground, keeping them straight.

- Open your legs wide, then cross one leg over the other in a scissor motion.

- Repeat the movement for several repetitions, engaging your core throughout.

- Ensure controlled and deliberate movements to maximize effectiveness.

Side Leg Raise

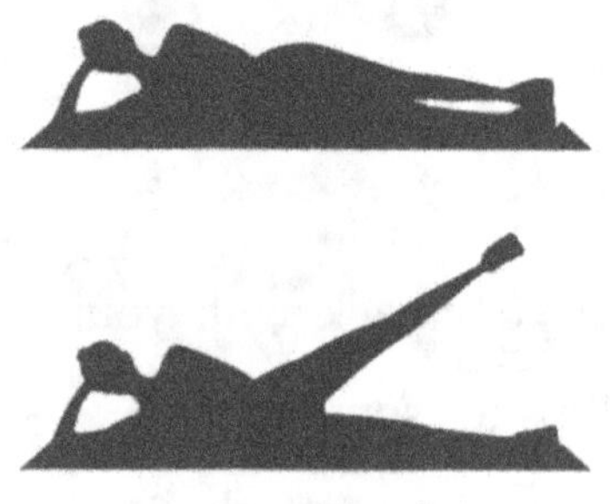

Side Leg Raise

- Lie on your side with your legs straight.
- Support your upper body with the head resting on your palm.
- Keep the other hand on your hip or in front of you.

- Lift the top leg as high as comfortably possible.
- Lower it back down without letting it touch the bottom leg.
- Repeat for the desired number of reps.
- Switch sides and repeat the process.

Lateral Side Leg Raises

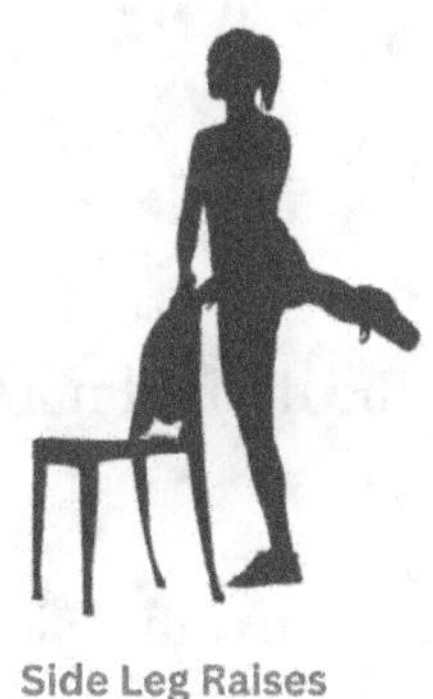

Side Leg Raises

- Stand upright with feet shoulder-width apart.
- Keep your core engaged for stability.

- Lift one leg directly to the side, keeping it straight.

- Use controlled movements to avoid swinging.

- Lift your leg to hip height or slightly higher.

- Focus on engaging the outer thigh muscles.

- Hold the raised position briefly, squeezing the muscles.

- Lower the leg back down slowly and with control.

- Perform the desired number of repetitions on one leg.

- Switch to the other leg and repeat the exercise.

Elbow to Opposite Knee

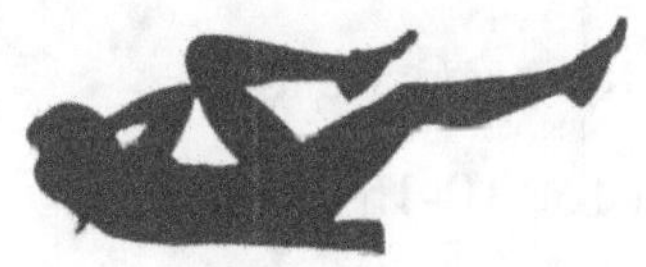

Elbow to Opposite Knee

- Start by lying on your back with your hands behind your head and your elbows pointing out.
- Lift your right elbow towards your left knee, engaging your core muscles.
- Simultaneously lift your left leg towards your right elbow, bringing them together diagonally.
- Hold the contraction momentarily, feeling the crunch in your abdominal muscles.

- Return to the starting position and repeat on the other side.

- Perform the exercise controlled, focusing on the connection between your elbow and the opposite knee.

- Aim for 10-15 repetitions on each side to target your obliques and improve core strength effectively

Chapter 7: Core Strengthening Balance Exercise

Modified Plank

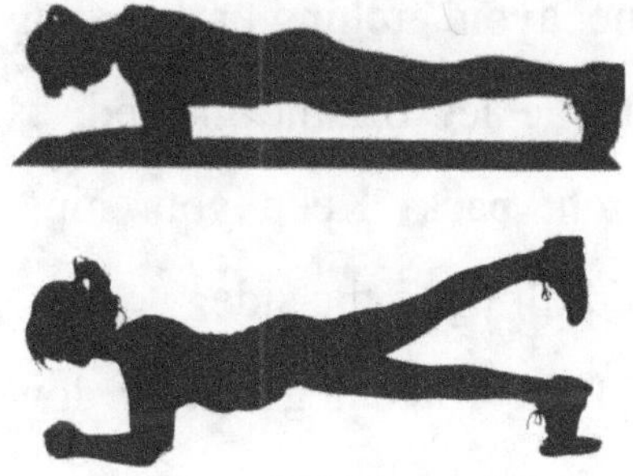

Modified Plank

- Begin on all fours with your hands directly beneath your shoulders and knees under your hips.

- Lower onto your forearms, keeping your elbows in line with your shoulders.

- Extend your legs behind you, toes on the ground, creating a straight line from head to heels.

- Tighten your core muscles by pulling your belly button toward your spine.

- Keep your back flat and maintain a neutral spine; avoid arching or rounding.

- Lift one leg off the ground, extending it straight back. Keep your hips level and avoid tilting to the side.

- Hold the lifted leg briefly, lower it back down, and switch to the other leg. Continue alternating legs throughout the exercise.

- Aim for holding the position for at least 20-30 seconds, gradually increasing as your strength improves.

Seated Leg Lifts

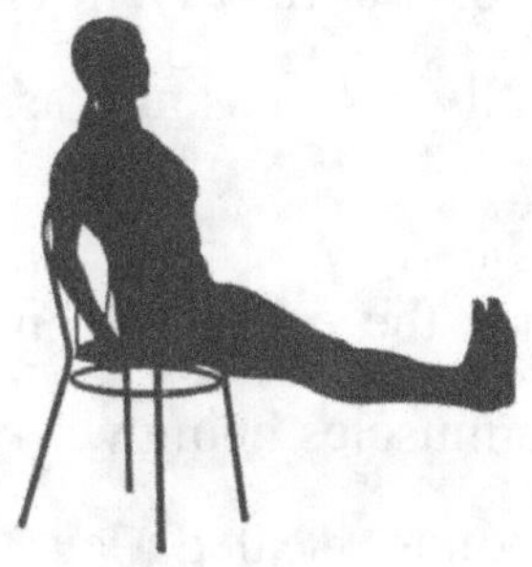

Seated Leg Lifts

- Sit on a sturdy chair with a straight back and feet flat on the floor.

- Hold onto the sides of the chair for support and stability.

- Lift the two legs straight out before you, keeping them extended and parallel to the ground.

- Hold the position for a few seconds, engaging your core and thigh muscles.

- Lower the legs back down to the starting position.

- Aim for 10-15 repetitions on each leg, gradually increasing as your strength improves.

- Perform the exercise controlled, focusing on the muscles being worked.

- Incorporate seated leg lifts into your regular workout routine for enhanced lower body strength and flexibility.

Superman

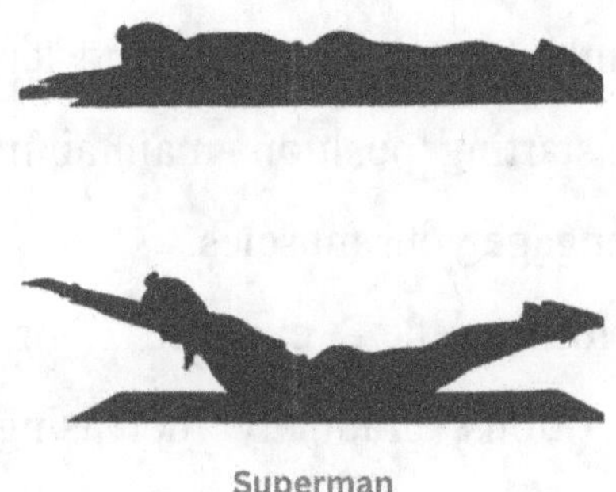

Superman

- Lie face down on a mat or the floor, with your arms extended straight before you.

- Tighten your core muscles, including your abs and lower back, to stabilize your spine.

- Simultaneously lift your arms, chest, and legs off the ground, keeping your neck neutral.

- Squeeze your glutes and lower back muscles as you lift, holding the position for a few seconds at the top.

- Gently lower your arms and legs back to the starting position, maintaining control to engage your muscles.

- Perform the exercise for several repetitions, gradually increasing as your strength improves.

Glute Bridge

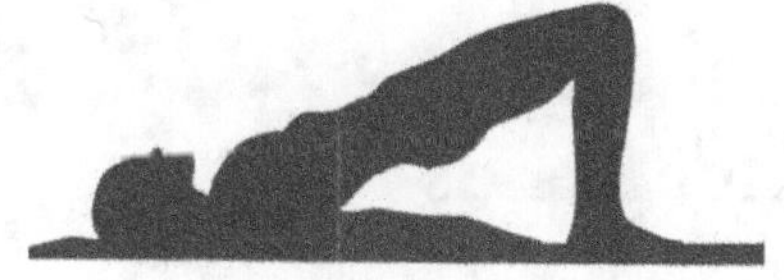

Glute Bridge

- Lie on your back with knees bent and feet flat, hip-width apart.
- Place your arms at your sides, palms facing down.
- Engage your core and squeeze your glutes as you lift your hips towards the ceiling.
- Form a straight line from shoulders to knees at the top, avoiding overextension.
- Hold for a moment, then lower your hips back down, almost touching the ground.

- Repeat for the desired number of repetitions, focusing on using your glutes to lift.

Seated Side Bends

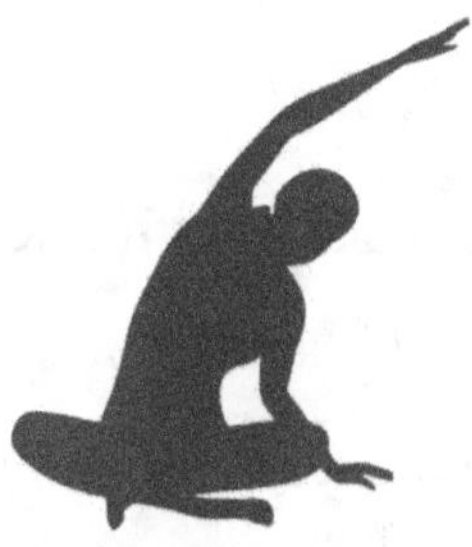

Seated Side Bends

- Begin comfortably seated (easy pose) with your legs crossed.
- Lower your left hand to the floor, ensuring a slight bend in your elbow for support.

- Extend your right arm upwards and over your head, gently leaning towards the left side.
- Feel the stretch along your right side, emphasizing the elongation of your torso.
- Maintain the position for 30 seconds to 1 minute, focusing on controlled breathing.
- Switch to the other side, placing your right hand on the floor and repeating the stretch.
- Engage your core for stability throughout the exercise.
- Gradually deepen the stretch as your flexibility improves over time.
- Perform 2-3 sets on each side, ensuring a smooth and controlled motion.

Seated Forward-Roll Up

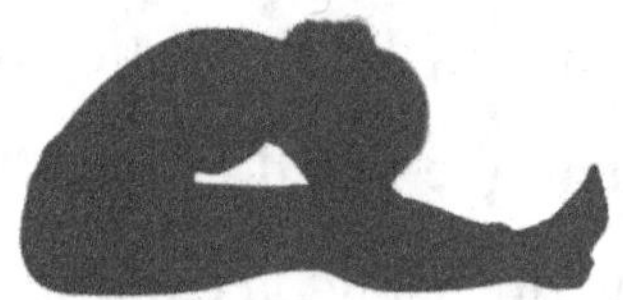

Seated Forward-Roll Up

- Start in a seated position, legs extended forward and flexed.
- Inhale, sitting tall with a straight spine.
- Exhale, hinge at the hips, maintaining spine length.
- Walk hands forward, stretching back and hamstrings.
- Flex feet, knees, and toes, pointing towards the ceiling.
- Inhale, lift and lengthen the chest slightly.

- Exhale and deepen the forward bend, allowing elbows to bend.
- Hold for 1-3 minutes, breathing consistently.
- To roll up back, release feet and slowly return to the seated position on an inhalation.

Forearm Plank

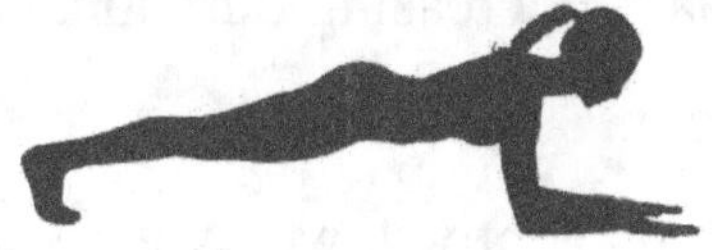

Forearm Plank

- Start on a yoga mat, positioning your elbows directly under your shoulders.
- Align your wrists with your elbows and spread your fingers wide for stability.
- Extend your legs straight behind you, resting on the balls of your feet.
- Keep your body straight from head to heels, engaging your core muscles.
- Ensure your hips are neither too high nor too low, maintaining a neutral spine.
- Gaze at the floor to avoid straining your neck, and breathe steadily.
- Hold the position for 20-60 seconds, gradually increasing duration as you build strength.
- To stop, gently lower your knees to the mat and rest in a child's pose.

Seated Half Roll-Backs

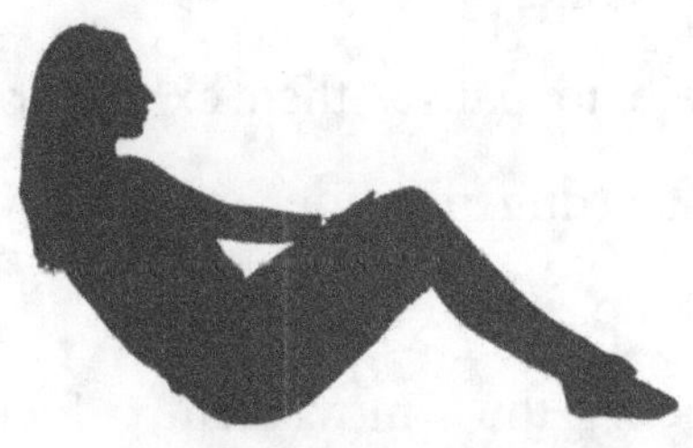

Seated Half Roll-Backs

- Sit on a mat with your knees bent and feet flat on the floor, hip-width apart.
- Place your hands at the back of your thighs, fingers pointing toward your knees.
- Inhale, engage your core, and lengthen your spine.
- Exhale, gently round your spine, and initiate the movement from your pelvis.

- Roll halfway back, keeping your core engaged and maintaining a C-curve in your spine.

- Inhale to pause, then exhale to return to the starting position, stacking your spine back up.

- Repeat the movement, focusing on controlled, fluid motions.

- Perform 8-10 repetitions, gradually increasing as your strength improves.

- Keep your shoulders relaxed and avoid straining your neck.

Triangle Pose

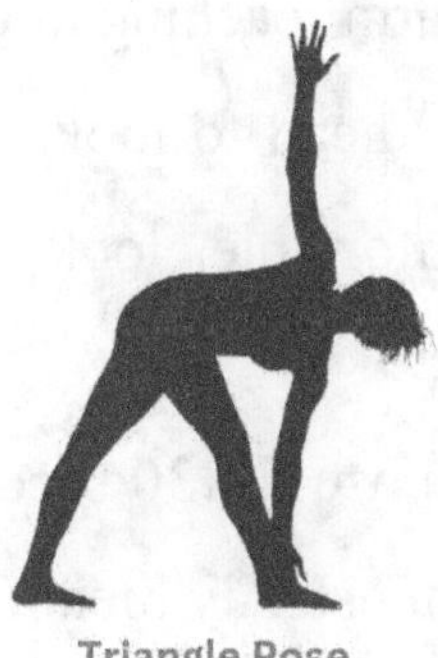

Triangle Pose

- Stand with your feet wide apart, parallel to each other

- Turn your right foot outward at a 90-degree angle and keep your left foot slightly inward.

- Extend your arms parallel to the floor, palms facing down.

- Shift your torso to the right and hinge at your right hip, reaching your right hand towards the floor.

- Lower your right hand to the shin, ankle, or the floor outside your right foot. Keep your left arm reaching upward.

- Turn your head to look at your left hand, or if comfortable, look straight ahead or upward.

- Hold the pose for 30 seconds to 1 minute, maintaining steady breathing.

Crunches

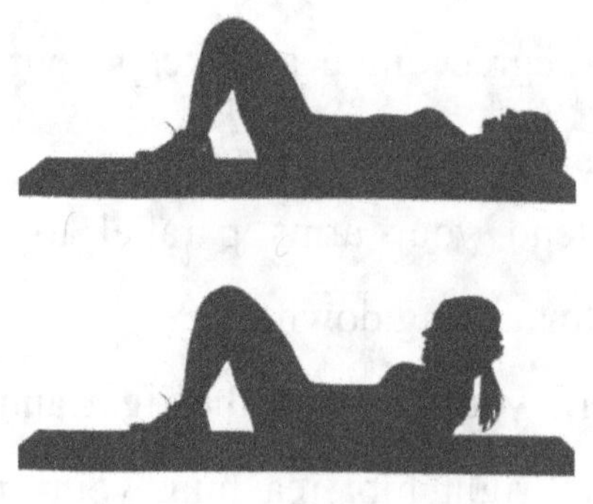

Crunches

- Lie on your back with your knees bent and feet flat on the floor.

- Place your hands gently behind your head, elbows pointing out.

- Inhale and engage your abdominal muscles by pulling your belly button towards your spine.

- Exhale as you lift your head, neck, and shoulders off the ground.

- Keep your gaze towards the ceiling, avoiding pulling on your neck.

- Feel the contraction in your abdominal muscles as you reach towards your knees.

- Inhale and slowly lower your upper body back to the starting position with control.

- Perform the exercise in a controlled manner for the desired number of repetitions.

- Aim for 2-3 sets of 15-20 crunches, gradually increasing as your strength improves.

Chapter 8: Stretching Exercise

Hamstring Stretches

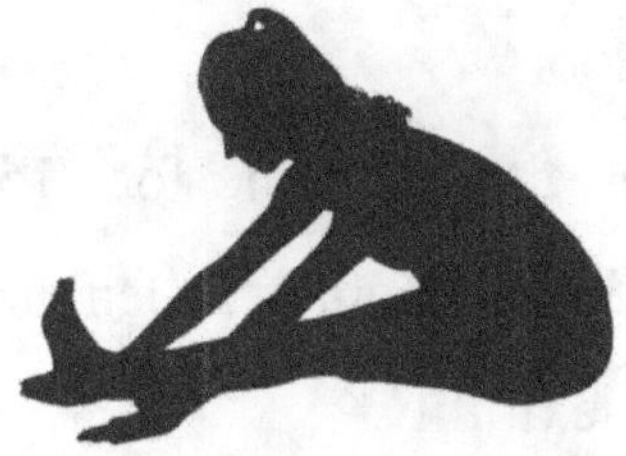

Hamstring Stretches

- Sit on the mat with your legs extended straight in front of you.
- Extend one leg outward while bending the other knee, bringing the sole of the foot to the inner thigh of the extended leg.

- Ensure your extended leg is straight, your toes point upward, and both hips are grounded on the floor.

- Hinge at your hips and lean forward from your waist, reaching toward your toes with both hands or placing your hands on the floor.

- Hold the stretch for 15-30 seconds, breathing deeply to enhance relaxation and flexibility.

- Repeat the stretch on the other leg by extending the opposite leg and bending the knee.

- Perform the stretch 2-3 times on each leg, gradually increasing the duration as your flexibility improves.

Triceps Stretches

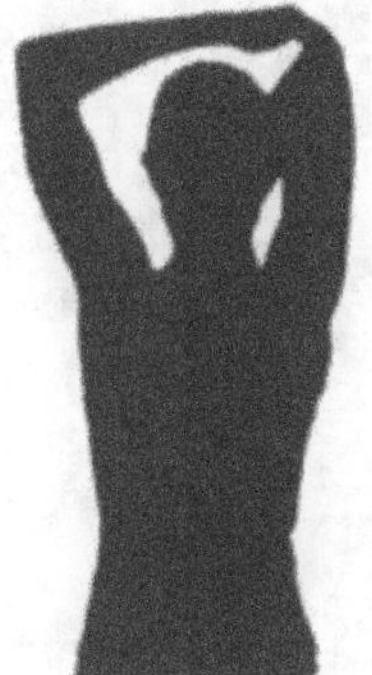

Triceps Stretches

- Stand or sit with a straight spine.

- Lift your right arm overhead, reaching towards the ceiling.

- Bend the right elbow, bringing your hand down the center of your back.

- Use your left hand to gently pat your right hand on your back, reaching for your fingertips.

- Feel the stretch in your triceps and the back of your arm.

- Maintain the stretch for 15-30 seconds, breathing deeply.
- Release the stretch and switch to the left arm, repeating the process.

Neck Stretches

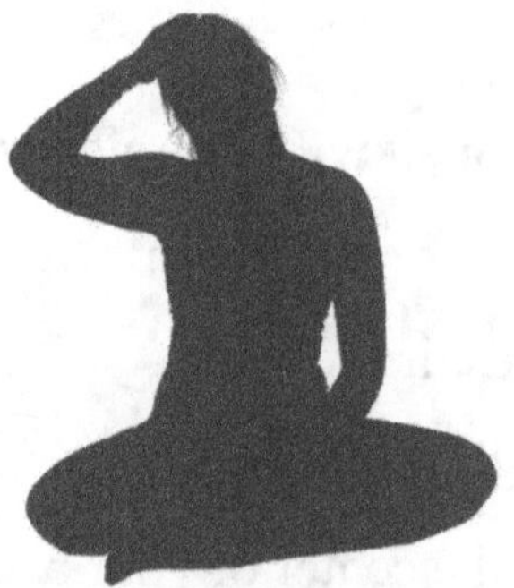

Neck Stretches

- Sit or stand comfortably with a straight spine.
- Drop your shoulders down, away from your ears.

- Gently lower your chin towards your chest.

- Slowly tilt your head to one side with the support of your hands, bringing your ear towards your shoulder. Hold for a few seconds.

- Rotate your head to one side, bringing your chin towards your shoulder. Hold the stretch.

- Repeat steps 4 and 5 on the other side for a balanced stretch.

Kneeling Hip Flexor Stretches

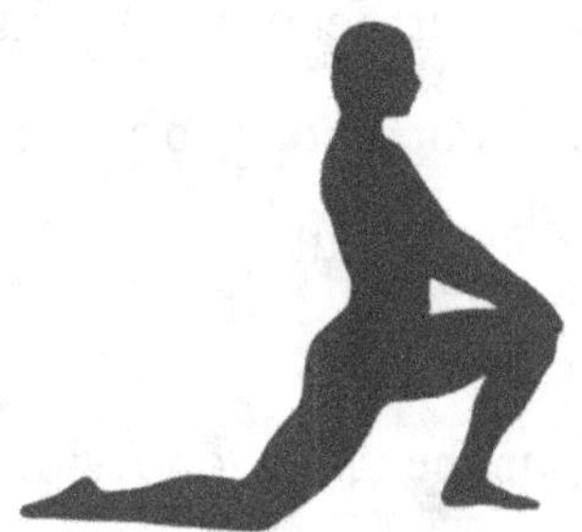

Kneeling Hip Flexor Stretches

- Start kneeling on both knees with your bottom on heels balls of feet against the mat.
- Lean forward, press palms to the mat, hands shoulder-width apart, and elbows slightly bent.
- Bring the left knee forward between arms, placing the left foot flat on the mat for a 90-degree angle.

- Straighten your upper body, placing both hands on the left knee for support.

- Extend the right leg behind you, the right knee on the mat, top of the right foot resting on the mat.

- Lean forward slightly to deepen the stretch, holding for 20-30 seconds.

- Release the stretch and repeat on the other side.

Shoulder Rolls

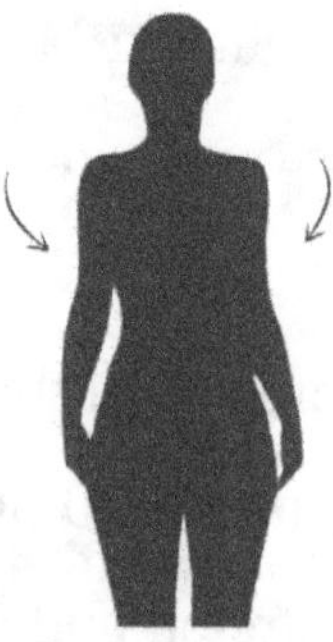

Shoulder Rolls

- Stand with your feet shoulder-width apart.

- Keep your arms relaxed by your sides.

- Inhale deeply as you lift your shoulders towards your ears.

- Exhale slowly as you roll your shoulders back and down in a circular motion.

- Repeat the shoulder rolls for 10-15 repetitions.

- Reverse the direction, rolling your shoulders forward for another 10-15 repetitions.

- Maintain a steady and controlled pace throughout the exercise.

- Focus on releasing tension and promoting flexibility in the shoulder muscles.

- Incorporate shoulder rolls into your warm-up routine or as a quick mid-day stretch.

Quadriceps Stretch

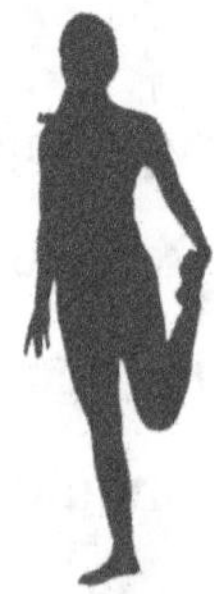

Quadriceps Stretch

- Stand upright with feet hip-width apart.
- Lift your right foot towards your buttocks, holding the ankle with your right hand.
- Keep your knees close together, pointing downwards.
- Engage your core to maintain balance.
- Hold the stretch for 15-30 seconds, feeling the stretch in the front of your thigh.
- Release and switch to the left leg.
- Repeat the stretch on both legs 2-3 times.

Chest Stretches

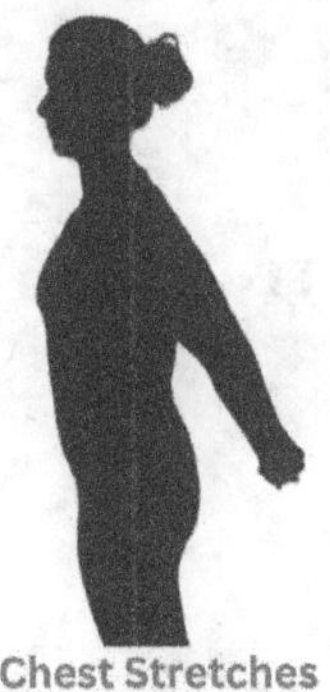

Chest Stretches

- Stand tall with feet shoulder-width apart.

- Extend your hands behind your back.

- Straighten your arms and lift them slightly.

- Open your chest by squeezing your shoulder blades together.

- Keep your head neutral and gaze forward.

- Hold the stretch for 15-30 seconds, breathing deeply.
- Release and repeat as needed for flexibility and posture improvement.

Lower Back Stretches

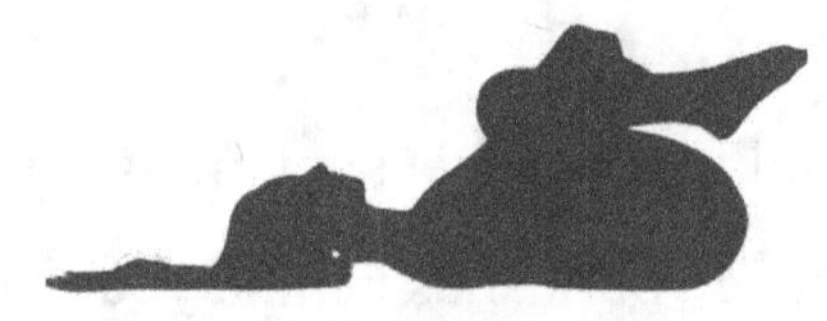

Lower Back Stretches

- Start by lying on your back with your knees bent and feet flat on the floor.
- Bring your two knees towards your chest, clasping your hands around it.

- Hold the stretch for 15-30 seconds, feeling a gentle pull in your lower back and buttocks.

- Return to the starting position with both knees bent.

- Cross your right ankle over your left knee, pulling the left knee towards your chest.

- Hold for 15-30 seconds, feeling the stretch in your right hip and lower back.

- Repeat the stretch on the other side by crossing your left ankle over your right knee.

- Aim for 2-3 sets on each side, gradually increasing the duration as your flexibility improves.

Cat-Cow Stretches

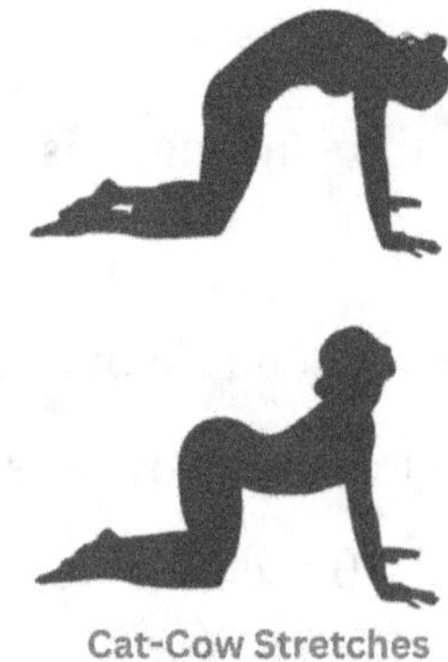

Cat-Cow Stretches

- Start in a tabletop position with hands beneath shoulders and knees under hips.

- Inhale, arch your back, dropping your belly towards the floor for the "cow" pose.

- Exhale and round your spine, tucking your chin to your chest for the "cat" pose.

- Repeat the sequence, flowing smoothly between cat and cow poses for a gentle spinal stretch.

- Coordinate movements with your breath, inhaling for the cow pose and exhaling for the cat pose.
- Continue for 1-2 minutes, focusing on the fluidity of the motion to enhance flexibility and release tension.

Calf Stretches

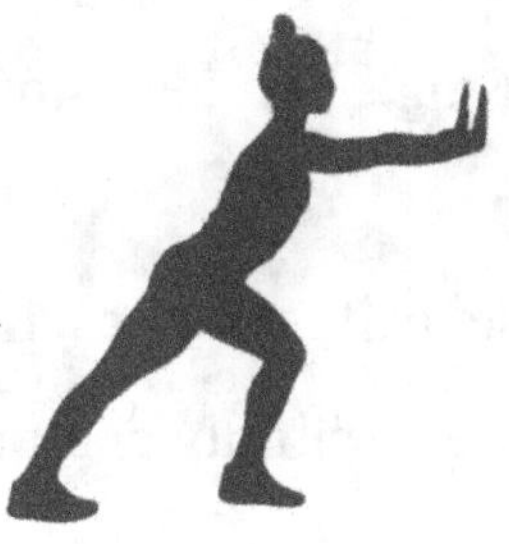

Calf Stretches

- Stand facing a wall with your hands resting on it at shoulder height.

- Step back with your right foot, keeping it straight, and bend your left knee slightly.

- Ensure your right heel is firmly on the ground and your toes are pointing forward.

- Lean forward, feeling the stretch in your right calf.

- Hold for 15-30 seconds, breathing deeply.

- Switch legs and repeat the stretch on the left side.

- Perform 2-3 sets on each leg, gradually increasing the duration for a deeper stretch.

- Include calf stretches in your routine to improve flexibility and prevent tightness.

Chapter 9: Conclusion

Prioritizing balance exercises for individuals aged 60 and beyond is crucial for maintaining overall well-being and preventing falls or injuries. By engaging in regular balance exercises, older adults can enhance their proprioception, coordination, and strength, contributing to better stability. This not only reduces the risk of falls but also promotes confidence and independence in daily activities.

Embracing a proactive mindset towards maintaining balance through targeted exercises is an investment in a vibrant and fulfilling later life. By incorporating these practices into daily routines, individuals in their 60s and beyond can not only preserve their physical health but also enhance their overall quality of life, ensuring

they continue to lead active and independent
lives.

Week_______________________

Monday Exercises:

Tuesday Exercises:

Wednesday Exercises:

Thursday Exercises:

Friday Exercises:

Saturday Exercises:

Sunday Exercises:

Month_______________________

Weekly Goals

- ☐ _______________________
- ☐ _______________________
- ☐ _______________________
- ☐ _______________________

My Motivation

Notes / Reminder

Week_________________________

Month___________________________

Monday Exercises:

Tuesday Exercises:

Wednesday Exercises:

Thursday Exercises:

Friday Exercises:

Saturday Exercises:

Sunday Exercises:

Weekly Goals

○ ☐ _______________________
○ ☐ _______________________
○ ☐ _______________________
○ ☐ _______________________

My Motivation

Notes / Reminder

Week______________________

Monday Exercises:

Tuesday Exercises:

Wednesday Exercises:

Thursday Exercises:

Friday Exercises:

Saturday Exercises:

Sunday Exercises:

Month______________________

Weekly Goals

- ☐ ____________________
- ☐ ____________________
- ☐ ____________________
- ☐ ____________________

My Motivation

Notes / Reminder

Week_______________________

Monday Exercises:

Tuesday Exercises:

Wednesday Exercises:

Thursday Exercises:

Friday Exercises:

Saturday Exercises:

Sunday Exercises:

Month_______________________

Weekly Goals

- ○ ☐ _______________________
- ○ ☐ _______________________
- ○ ☐ _______________________
- ○ ☐ _______________________

My Motivation

Notes / Reminder

Week__________________________

Month__________________________

Monday Exercises:

Tuesday Exercises:

Wednesday Exercises:

Thursday Exercises:

Friday Exercises:

Saturday Exercises:

Sunday Exercises:

Weekly Goals

My Motivation

Notes / Reminder

Week______________________

Month______________________

Monday Exercises:

Tuesday Exercises:

Wednesday Exercises:

Thursday Exercises:

Friday Exercises:

Saturday Exercises:

Sunday Exercises:

Weekly Goals

- ○ ☐ __________________
- ○ ☐ __________________
- ○ ☐ __________________
- ○ ☐ __________________

My Motivation

Notes / Reminder

Week________________________

Month________________________

Monday Exercises:

Tuesday Exercises:

Wednesday Exercises:

Thursday Exercises:

Friday Exercises:

Saturday Exercises:

Sunday Exercises:

Weekly Goals

- ⊙ ☐ ________________________
- ⊙ ☐ ________________________
- ⊙ ☐ ________________________
- ⊙ ☐ ________________________

My Motivation

Notes / Reminder

Week________________________

Month________________________

Monday Exercises:

Tuesday Exercises:

Wednesday Exercises:

Thursday Exercises:

Friday Exercises:

Saturday Exercises:

Sunday Exercises:

Weekly Goals

- ☐ ________________________
- ☐ ________________________
- ☐ ________________________
- ☐ ________________________

My Motivation

Notes / Reminder

Week_______________________

Monday Exercises:

Tuesday Exercises:

Wednesday Exercises:

Thursday Exercises:

Friday Exercises:

Saturday Exercises:

Sunday Exercises:

Month_______________________

Weekly Goals

- ⦿ ☐ _______________________
- ⦿ ☐ _______________________
- ⦿ ☐ _______________________
- ⦿ ☐ _______________________

My Motivation

Notes / Reminder

Week_____________________

Monday Exercises:

Tuesday Exercises:

Wednesday Exercises:

Thursday Exercises:

Friday Exercises:

Saturday Exercises:

Sunday Exercises:

Month_____________________

Weekly Goals

○ ☐ _______________________
○ ☐ _______________________
○ ☐ _______________________
○ ☐ _______________________

My Motivation

Notes / Reminder

Week_____________________

Month_____________________

Monday Exercises:

Tuesday Exercises:

Wednesday Exercises:

Thursday Exercises:

Friday Exercises:

Saturday Exercises:

Sunday Exercises:

Weekly Goals

- ☐ _______________
- ☐ _______________
- ☐ _______________
- ☐ _______________

My Motivation

Notes / Reminder

Week_________________   Month___________________________

| Monday Exercises: | **Weekly Goals** |

Monday Exercises:

Tuesday Exercises:

Wednesday Exercises:

Thursday Exercises:

Friday Exercises:

Saturday Exercises:

Sunday Exercises:

Weekly Goals

- ○ ☐ _______________________
- ○ ☐ _______________________
- ○ ☐ _______________________
- ○ ☐ _______________________

My Motivation

Notes / Reminder

Week________________

Month________________

Monday Exercises:

Tuesday Exercises:

Wednesday Exercises:

Thursday Exercises:

Friday Exercises:

Saturday Exercises:

Sunday Exercises:

Weekly Goals

- ⦿ ☐ ________________
- ⦿ ☐ ________________
- ⦿ ☐ ________________
- ⦿ ☐ ________________

My Motivation

Notes / Reminder

Week_____________________

Month_____________________

Monday Exercises:

Tuesday Exercises:

Wednesday Exercises:

Thursday Exercises:

Friday Exercises:

Saturday Exercises:

Sunday Exercises:

Weekly Goals

- ☐ _______________________
- ☐ _______________________
- ☐ _______________________
- ☐ _______________________

My Motivation

Notes / Reminder

Week________________________

Monday Exercises:

Tuesday Exercises:

Wednesday Exercises:

Thursday Exercises:

Friday Exercises:

Saturday Exercises:

Sunday Exercises:

Month________________________

Weekly Goals

- ☐ ________________________
- ☐ ________________________
- ☐ ________________________
- ☐ ________________________

My Motivation

Notes / Reminder

Week_________________________

Monday Exercises:

Tuesday Exercises:

Wednesday Exercises:

Thursday Exercises:

Friday Exercises:

Saturday Exercises:

Sunday Exercises:

Month_____________________________

Weekly Goals

- ○ ☐ _________________________
- ○ ☐ _________________________
- ○ ☐ _________________________
- ○ ☐ _________________________

My Motivation

Notes / Reminder

Week_______________________

Month_______________________

Monday Exercises:

Tuesday Exercises:

Wednesday Exercises:

Thursday Exercises:

Friday Exercises:

Saturday Exercises:

Sunday Exercises:

Weekly Goals

- ☐ _______________________
- ☐ _______________________
- ☐ _______________________
- ☐ _______________________

My Motivation

Notes / Reminder

Week_______________________

Monday Exercises:

Tuesday Exercises:

Wednesday Exercises:

Thursday Exercises:

Friday Exercises:

Saturday Exercises:

Sunday Exercises:

Month_______________________

Weekly Goals

- ⚪ ☐ _______________________
- ⚪ ☐ _______________________
- ⚪ ☐ _______________________
- ⚪ ☐ _______________________

My Motivation

Notes / Reminder

Week______________________

Month______________________

Monday Exercises:

Tuesday Exercises:

Wednesday Exercises:

Thursday Exercises:

Friday Exercises:

Saturday Exercises:

Sunday Exercises:

Weekly Goals

- ☐ ______________________
- ☐ ______________________
- ☐ ______________________
- ☐ ______________________

My Motivation

Notes / Reminder

Week______________________

Monday Exercises:

Tuesday Exercises:

Wednesday Exercises:

Thursday Exercises:

Friday Exercises:

Saturday Exercises:

Sunday Exercises:

Month______________________

Weekly Goals

- ☐ _______________________
- ☐ _______________________
- ☐ _______________________
- ☐ _______________________

My Motivation

Notes / Reminder

Week______________________

Monday Exercises:

Tuesday Exercises:

Wednesday Exercises:

Thursday Exercises:

Friday Exercises:

Saturday Exercises:

Sunday Exercises:

Month______________________

Weekly Goals

- ○ ☐ ___________________
- ○ ☐ ___________________
- ○ ☐ ___________________
- ○ ☐ ___________________

My Motivation

Notes / Reminder

www.ingramcontent.com/pod-product-compliance
Lightning Source LLC
Chambersburg PA
CBHW071221260726
48653CB00042B/1482